Easy Keto Slow Cooker Cookbook

50 Super Easy And Stress-Free Ketogenic Recipes

Elena Johnson

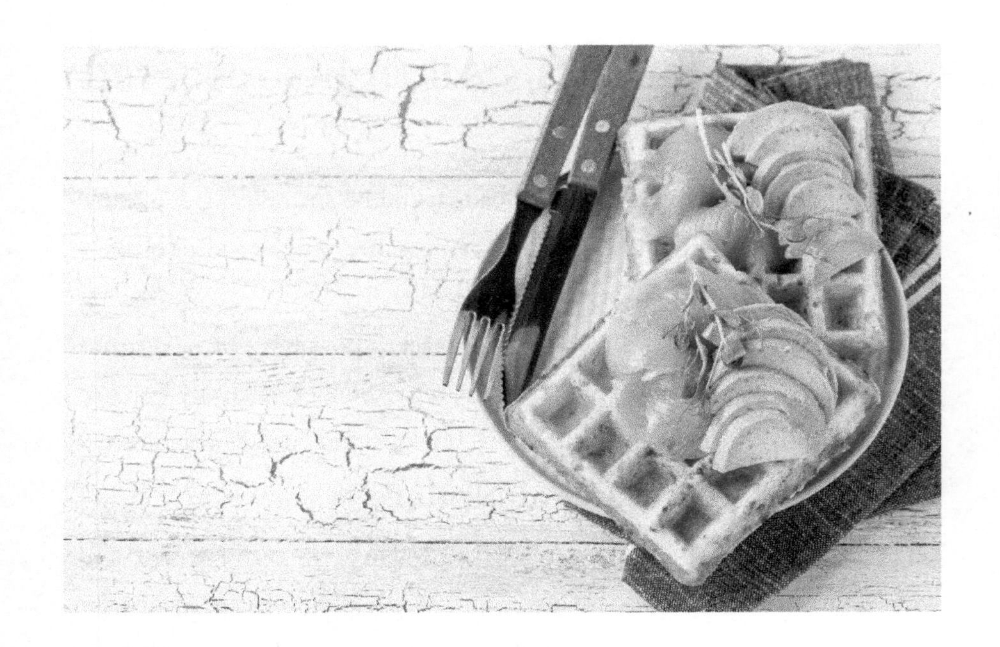

TABLE OF CONTENTS

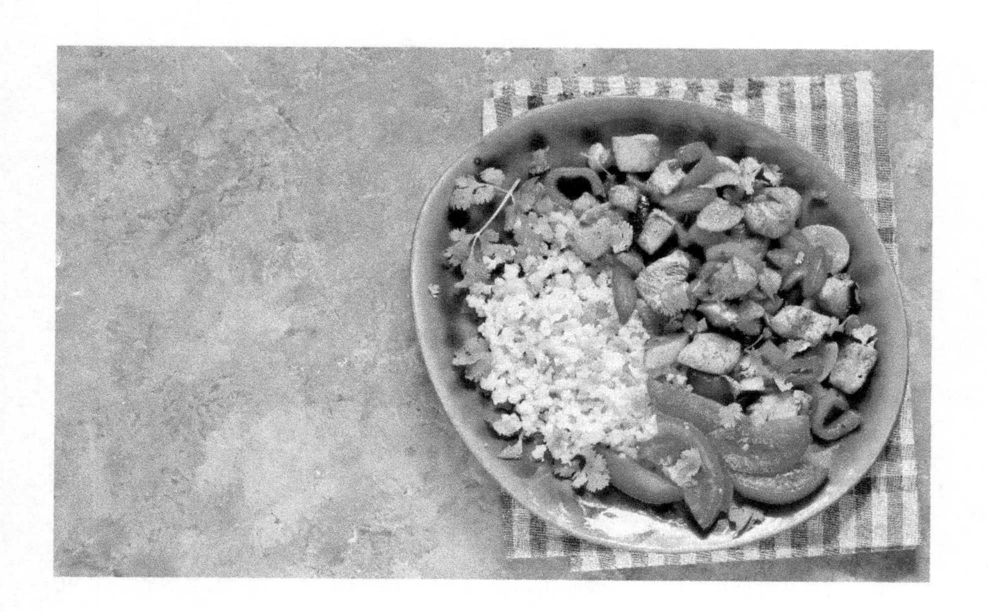

INTRODUCTION

The ketogenic diet is trendy, and for an excellent reason. It truly teaches healthy eating without forcing anyone into at risk. The success rate of keto is relatively high. While there are no specific numbers to suggest the exact rate, it is only fair to state that those who have the will to change their lifestyle and are okay adjusting to new eating habits, almost every one of them will make it through as a success story.

A diet that results in the production of ketone bodies by the liver is called a ketogenic diet; it causes your system to use fat instead of carbohydrates for energy. Limit your carbohydrate intake to a low level, causing some reactions. However, it is not a high protein diet. It involves moderate protein, low carbohydrate intake, and high fat intake.

Regardless of your lifestyle, everyone benefits from the keto diet in the following ways:

Weight Loss

Far more important than the visual aspect of excess weight is its negative influence on your body. Too much weight affects the efficiency of your body's blood flow, which in turn also affects how much oxygen your heart is able to pump to every part of your system. Too much weight also means that there are layers of fat covering your internal organs, which prevents them from working efficiently. It makes it hard to walk because it puts great pressure on your joints, and makes it very difficult to complete even regular daily tasks. A healthy weight allows your body to move freely and your entire internal system to work at its optimal levels.

Cognitive Focus

In order for your brain to function at its best, it needs to have balanced levels of all nutrients and molecules, because a balance allows it to focus on other things, such as working, studying, or creativity. If you eat carbs, the sudden insulin spike that comes with them will force your brain to stop whatever it was doing and to turn its focus on the correct breakdown of glucose molecules. This is why people often feel sleepy and with a foggy mind after high-carb meals. The keto diet keeps the balance strong, so that your brain does not have to deal with any sudden surprises.

Blood Sugar Control

If you already have diabetes, or are prone to it, then controlling your blood sugar is obviously of the utmost importance. However, even if you are not battling a type of diabetes at the moment, that doesn't mean that you are not in danger of developing it in the future. Most people forget that insulin is a finite resource in your body. You are given a certain amount of it, and it is gradually used up throughout your life. The more often you eat carbs, the more often your body needs to use insulin to break down the glucose; and when it reaches critically low levels of this finite resource, diabetes is formed.

Lower Cholesterol and Blood Pressure

Cholesterol and triglyceride levels maintain, or ruin, your arterial health. If your arteries are clogged up with cholesterol, they cannot efficiently transfer blood through your system, which in some cases even results in heart attacks. The keto diet keeps all of these levels at an optimal level, so that they do not interfere with your body's normal functioning.

Slow Cookers

Slow cookers are not new appliances in the culinary world. They have been around for decades; you might even have fond memories from your childhood of your parents serving your favorite dinner out of one. Slow cookers are very versatile because the cooking environment works the same no matter the cuisine. Knowing what slow cookers can and can't do is important for planning your meals, especially for a diet like keto.

Some of the reasons to use a slow cooker include:

Enhances flavor: Cooking ingredients over several hours with spices, herbs, and other seasonings creates vegetables and proteins that burst with delicious flavors. This slow process allows the flavors to mellow and deepen for an enhanced eating experience.

Saves time: Cooking at home takes a great deal of time: prepping, sautéing, stirring, turning the heat up and down, and watching the meal so that it does not over- or undercook. If you're unable to invest the time, you might find yourself reaching for convenience foods instead of healthy choices. Slow cookers allow you to do other activities while the meal cooks. You can put your ingredients in the slow cooker in the morning and come home to a perfectly cooked meal.

Convenient: Besides the time-saving aspect, using a slow cooker can free up the stove and oven for other dishes. This can be very convenient for large holiday meals or when you want to serve a side dish and entrée as well as a delectable dessert. Clean up is simple when you use the slow cooker for messy meals because most inserts are nonstick or are easily cleaned with a little soapy water, and each meal is prepared in either just the machine or using one additional vessel to sauté ingredients. There is no wide assortment of pots, pans, and baking dishes to contend with at the end of the day.

Low heat production: If you have ever cooked dinner on a scorching summer afternoon, you will appreciate the low amount of heat produced by a slow cooker. Even after eight hours of operation, slow cookers do not heat up your kitchen and you will not be sweating over the hot stovetop. Slow cookers use about a third of the energy of conventional cooking methods, just a little more energy than a traditional light bulb.

Supports healthy eating: Cooking your food at high heat can reduce the nutrition profile of your foods, breaking down and removing the majority of vitamins, minerals, and antioxidants while producing unhealthy chemical compounds that can contribute to disease. Low-heat cooking retains all the goodness that you want for your diet.

Saves Money: Slow cookers save you money because of the low amount of electricity they use and because the best ingredients for slow cooking are the less expensive cuts of beef and heartier inexpensive vegetables. Tougher cuts of meat—brisket, chuck, shanks—break down beautifully to fork-tender goodness. Another cost-saving benefit is that most 6-quart slow cookers will produce enough of a recipe to stretch your meals over at least two days. Leftovers are one of the best methods for saving money.

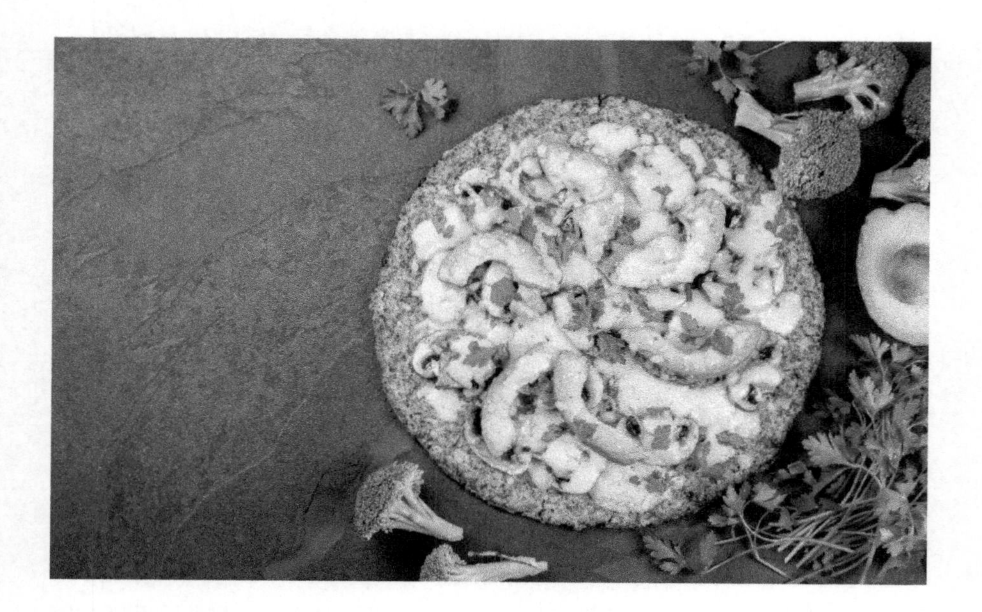

BREAKFAST

1. Kale, Bacon, and Cheese Breakfast Casserole

Preparation Time: 5 minutes   Cooking Time: 4 hours

Servings: 6

Ingredients:

- 1large kale, chopped
- 1tbsp.. olive oil
- cup four cheese mix, grated
- 10 eggs, beaten
- Salt and pepper to taste

Directions:

1. Mix all ingredients in a bowl.
2. Place inside the freezer.
3. Once you are ready to cook the meal, allow thawing on the countertop for at least 2 hours.
4. Place all ingredients in the Crock-Pot. Cook on high

Nutrition: Calories: 352 Carbohydrates: 2.5 g Protein: 26.2 g Fat: 35.1 g Sugar: 0.3 g Sodium: 521 mg Fiber: 1.4 g

2. Egg Casserole with Italian Cheeses, Sun-Dried Tomatoes, and Herbs

Preparation Time: 5 minutes

Cooking Time: 4 hours

Servings: 8

Ingredients:

- 10eggs
- 2tbsp.. milk
- 3tbsp.. sun-dried tomatoes, chopped
- 2tbsp.. onion, minced
- 2tbsp.. basil, chopped
- 1tbsp.. thyme leaves
- Salt and pepper to taste
- 1cup mixed Italian cheeses, grated

Directions:

1. Mix all ingredients in a bowl.
2. Place inside the freezer.
3. Once you are ready to cook the meal, allow thawing on the countertop for at least 2 hours.
4. Place all ingredients in the Crock-Pot.

5. Cook on high

Nutrition: Calories: 140 Carbohydrates: 3.87 g Protein: 10.93 g Fat: 8.89 g Sugar: 1.27 g Sodium: 309 mg Fiber: 0.3 g

3. Egg and Cheese Casserole with Chayote Squash

Preparation Time: 5 minutes

Cooking Time: 4 hours

Servings: 6

Ingredients:

- 1tsp.. olive oil
- 1red onion, diced
- 2 small chayote squash, grated
- 1/2 small red bell pepper, diced
- 10 large eggs, beaten
- 1/4 cup low-fat cottage cheese
- 2tbsp.. milk
- 1/2tsp.. ground cumin
- 2cups grated cheese
- Salt and pepper to taste

Directions:

1. Combine all ingredients in a mixing bowl.
2. Place inside the freezer.
3. Once you are ready to cook the meal, allow thawing on the countertop for at least 2 hours.

4. Pour into the Crock-Pot.
5. Close and cook on high

Nutrition: Calories: 409 Carbohydrates: 3.6 g Protein: 35.2 g Fat: 33.6 g Sugar: 1.5 g Sodium: 362 mg Fiber: 3.2 g

4. Sausage and Kale Strata

Time: 5 minutes Cooking Time: 4 hours Servings: 12

Ingredients:

- 12 eggs, beaten
- 2 1/2 cups milk
- Salt and pepper to taste
- 2 tbsp.. fresh oregano, minced
- 2 lb.. breakfast sausages, sliced
- bunch kale, torn into pieces
- 16 oz.. white mushrooms, sliced
- 2 1/2 cups cheese,

Directions:

1. Combine all ingredients
2. Place inside the freezer.
3. Once you are ready to cook the meal, allow thawing on the countertop for at least 2 hours.
4. Pour the ingredients into the Crock-Pot and close the lid. Cook on high .

Nutrition: Calories: 431 Carbohydrates: 4.5 g Protein: 32.3 g Fat: 37.4 g Sugar: 0.6 g Sodium: 525 mg Fiber: 3.2 g

5. Egg Cake Recipe with Peppers, Kale, and Cheddar

Preparation Time: 10 minutes

Cooking Time: 4 hours

Servings: 6

Ingredients:

- 1doz.en eggs, beaten
- 1/4 cup milk
- 1/4 cup almond flour
- clove garlic, minced
- Salt and pepper to taste
- 1 cup kale, chopped
- red bell pepper, chopped
- 3/4 cup mozzarella cheese, grated
- 1 green onion, chopped

Directions:

1. In a mixing bowl, combine all ingredients.
2. Place inside the freezer.
3. Once you are ready to cook the meal, allow thawing on the countertop for at least 2 hours.
4. Pour the ingredients into the Crock-Pot and close the lid.

5. Close and cook on high .

Nutrition: Calories: 527 Carbohydrates: 3.1 g Protein: 42.3 g Fat: 45.6 g Sugar: 0.5 g Sodium: 425 mg Fiber: 2.4 g

6. Feta Cheese and Kale Breakfast Casserole

Preparation Time: 5 minutes

Cooking Time: 4 hours

Servings: 6

Ingredients:

- 10oz.. kale, chopped
- 2tsp.s. olive oil
- 3/4 cup feta cheese, crumbled
- 12 eggs, beaten
- Salt and pepper to taste

Directions:

1. Combine all ingredients.
2. Place inside the freezer.
3. Once you are ready to cook the meal, allow thawing on the countertop for at least 2 hours.
4. Pour the ingredients into the Crock-Pot and close the lid.
5. Cook on high .

Nutrition: Calories: 397 Carbohydrates: 4 g Protein: 32.2 g Fat: 29.4 g Sugar: 0.6 g Sodium: 425 mg Fiber: 3.2 g

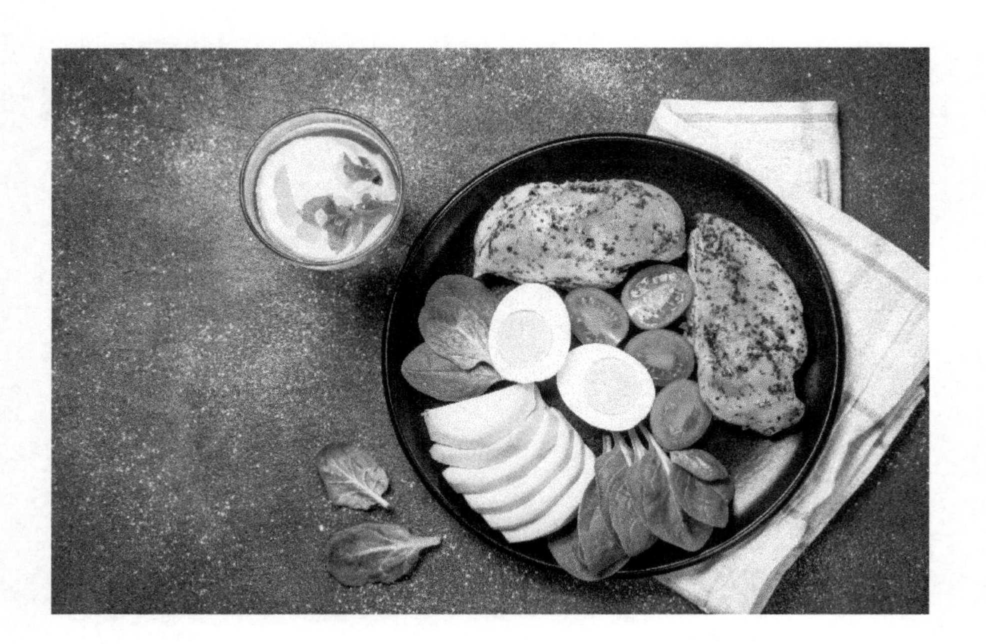

LUNCH

7. Chicken and Broccoli

Preparation time: 10 minutes

Cooking time: 6 hours

Servings: 6

Ingredients:

- 1cup chicken broth
- 1/2cup oyster sauce
- 1/4cup tamari or low-sodium soy sauce
- 1/4cup (packed) brown sugar
- 1teaspoon toasted sesame oil
- 1teaspoon garlic powder
- 2pounds boneless, skinless chicken thighs, trimmed of excess fat and cut into bite-size pieces
- 2tablespoons cornstarch
- 2tablespoons water
- 1(16-ounce) package froz.en broccoli florets

Directions:

1. Combine the chicken broth, oyster sauce, tamari, brown sugar, sesame oil, and garlic powder in the slow cooker. Whisk until smooth. Add the chicken pieces and stir to coat with the sauce.
2. Cover and cook on low for 6 hours, or until the chicken is tender.
3. Remove the lid and turn the cooker to high. Make a cornstarch slurry by whisking the cornstarch and water together in a small bowl. Add the slurry to the liquid in the slow cooker and whisk until dissolved.
4. Pour the broccoli into a colander. Run hot water over the broccoli until it's warmed through. Shake off the excess water and then stir the broccoli into the slow cooker. Cover and cook on high for 10 minutes, or until the broccoli is cooked through and the sauce is thickened by the cornstarch. Serve.

Nutrition: Calories 213, Fat 11, Fiber 13 Carbs 3.8 Protein 23

8. Honey-Garlic Chicken

Preparation time: 10 minutes Cooking time: 6 hours

Servings: 6-8

Ingredients:

- 2pounds boneless or bone-in, skinless chicken thighs, trimmed of excess fat
- 1/4cup all-purpose flour
- 1/3cup honey
- 1/3cup tamari or low-sodium soy sauce
- 1/3cup fresh lemon juice
- 1tablespoon instant tapioca
- 2teaspoons garlic powder

Directions:

1. Dredge the chicken thighs in the flour and put them in the slow cooker.
2. In a small bowl, whisk together the honey, tamari, lemon juice, tapioca, and garlic powder. Pour the sauce over the chicken.
3. Cover and cook on low for 6 hours, or until the chicken is tender. Serve the chicken with the sauce.

Nutrition: Calories 365, Fat 13, Fiber 9 Carbs 3.6 Protein 12

9. Aromatic Jalapeno Wings

Preparation time: 10 minutes

Cooking time: 3 hours

Servings: 4

Ingredients:

- 1jalapeño pepper, diced
- 1/2cup of fresh cilantro, diced
- 3tablespoon of coconut oil
- Juice from 1 lime
- 2garlic cloves, peeled and minced
- Salt and black pepper ground, to taste
- 2lb. chicken wings
- Lime wedges, to serve
- Mayonnaise, to serve

Directions:

1. Start by throwing all the Ingredients into the large bowl and mix well.
2. Cover the wings and marinate them in the refrigerator for 2 hours.
3. Now add the wings along with their marinade into the Slow cooker.
4. Cover it and cook for 3 hours on Low Settings.

5. Garnish as desired.

6. Serve warm.

Nutrition: Calories 246 Fat 7.4 g Carbs 4 g Sugar 6.5 g Fiber 2.7 g Protein 37.2 g

10. Barbeque Chicken Wings

Preparation time: 10 minutes

Cooking time: 3 hours

Servings: 4

Ingredients:

- 2lb. chicken wings
- 1/2cup of water
- 1/2teaspoon of basil, dried
- 3/4cup of BBQ sauce
- 1/2cup of lime juice
- 1teaspoon of red pepper, crushed
- 2teaspoons of paprika
- 1/2cup of swerve
- Salt and black pepper- to taste
- A pinch cayenne peppers

Directions:

1. Start by throwing all the Ingredients into the Slow cooker and mix them well.
2. Cover it and cook for 3 hours on Low Settings.
3. Garnish as desired.

4. Serve warm.

Nutrition: Calories 457 Fat 19.1 g Carbs 3.9 g Sugar 1.2 g Fiber 1.7 g Protein 32.5 g

11. Saucy Duck

Preparation time: 10 minutes

Cooking time: 6 hours

Servings: 4

Ingredients

- 1duck, cut into small chunks
- 4garlic cloves, minced
- 4tablespoons of swerves
- 2green onions, roughly diced
- 4tablespoon of soy sauce
- 4tablespoon of sherry wine
- 1/4cup of water
- 1-inch ginger root, sliced
- A pinch salt
- black pepper to taste

Directions:

1. Start by throwing all the Ingredients into the Slow cooker and mix them well.
2. Cover it and cook for 6 hours on Low Settings.
3. Garnish as desired.

4. Serve warm.

Nutrition: Calories 338 Fat 3.8 g Carbs 3 g Fiber 2.4 g Sugar 1.2 g Protein 15.4g

12. Chicken Roux Gumbo

Preparation time: 10 minutes

Cooking time: 6 hours

Servings: 24

Ingredients:

- 1lb.. chicken thighs, cut into halves
- 1tablespoon of vegetable oil
- 1lb.. smoky sausage, sliced, crispy, and crumbled.
- Salt and black pepper- to taste
- Aromatics
- 1bell pepper, diced
- 2quarts' chicken stock
- 15oz.. canned tomatoes, diced
- 1celery stalk, diced
- salt to taste
- 2garlic cloves, minced
- 1/2lb. okra, sliced
- 1yellow onion, diced
- a dash Tabasco sauce
- For the roux:

- 1/2cup of almond flour
- 1/4cup of vegetable oil
- 1teaspoon of Cajun spice

Directions:

1. Start by throwing all the Ingredients except okra and roux Ingredients into the Slow cooker.
2. Cover it and cook for 5 hours on Low Settings.
3. Stir in okra and cook for another 1 hour on low heat.
4. Mix all the roux Ingredients and add them to the Slow cooker.
5. Stir cook on high heat until the sauce thickens.
6. Garnish as desired.
7. Serve warm.

Nutrition: Calories 604 Fat 30.6 g Carbs 1.4g Fiber 0.2 g Sugar 20.3 g Protein 54.6 g

13. Cider-Braised Chicken

Preparation time: 10 minutes

Cooking time: 5 hours

Servings: 2

Ingredients:

- 4chicken drumsticks
- 2tablespoon of olive oil
- 1/2cup of apple cider vinegar
- 1tablespoon of balsamic vinegar
- 1chili pepper, diced
- 1yellow onion, minced
- Salt and black pepper- to taste

Directions:

1. Start by throwing all the Ingredients into a bowl and mix them well.
2. Marinate this chicken for 2 hours in the refrigerator.
3. Spread the chicken along with its marinade in the Slow cooker.
4. Cover it and cook for 5 hours on Low Settings.
5. Garnish as desired. Serve warm.

Nutrition: Calories 311 Fat 25.5 g Carbs 1.4 g Fiber 0.7 g Sugar 0.3 g Protein 18.4 g

14. Chunky Chicken Salsa

Preparation time: 10 minutes

Cooking time: 6 hours

Servings: 2

Ingredients

- 1lb. chicken breast, skinless and boneless
- 1cup of chunky salsa
- 3/4teaspoon of cumin
- A pinch oregano
- Salt and black pepper- to taste

Directions:

1. Start by throwing all the Ingredients into the Slow cooker and mix them well.
2. Cover it and cook for 6 hours on Low Settings. Garnish as desired.
3. Serve warm.

Nutrition: Calories 541 Fat 34 g Carbs 3.4 g Fiber 1.2 g Sugar 1 g Protein 20.3 g

15. Dijon Chicken

Preparation time: 10 minutes

Cooking time: 6 hours

Servings: 4

Ingredients:

- 2lb. chicken thighs, skinless and boneless
- 3/ cup of chicken stock
- 1/4cup of lemon juice
- 2tablespoon of extra virgin olive oil
- 3tablespoon of Dijon mustard
- 2tablespoons of Italian seasoning
- Salt and black pepper- to taste

Directions:

1. Start by throwing all the Ingredients into the Slow cooker and mix them well.
2. Cover it and cook for 6 hours on Low Settings.
3. Garnish as desired.
4. Serve warm.

Nutrition: Calories 398 Fat 13.8 g Carbs 3.6 g Fiber 1 g Sugar 1.3 g Protein 51.8 g

16. Chicken Thighs with Vegetables

Preparation time: 10 minutes

Cooking time: 6 hours

Servings: 6

Ingredients:

- 6chicken thighs
- 1teaspoon of vegetable oil
- 15oz. canned tomatoes, diced
- 1yellow onion, diced
- 2tablespoon of tomato paste
- 1/2cup of white wine
- 2cups of chicken stock
- 1celery stalk, diced
- 1/4lb. baby carrots, cut into halves
- 1/2teaspoon of thyme, dried
- Salt and black pepper- to taste

Directions:

1. Start by throwing all the Ingredients into the Slow cooker and mix them well.
2. Cover it and cook for 6 hours on Low Settings.

3. Shred the slow-cooked chicken using a fork and return to the pot.
4. Mix well and garnish as desired.
5. Serve warm.

Nutrition: Calories 372 Fat 11.8 g Carbs 1.8 g Fiber 0.6 g Sugar 27.3 g Protein 34 g

17. Chicken dipped in tomatillo Sauce

Preparation time: 10 minutes

Cooking time: 6 hours

Servings: 4

Ingredients:

- 1lb. chicken thighs, skinless and boneless
- 2tablespoon of extra virgin olive oil
- 1yellow onion, sliced
- 1garlic clove, crushed
- 4oz. canned green chilies, diced
- 1handful cilantro, diced
- 15oz. cauliflower rice, already cooked
- 5oz. tomatoes, diced
- 15oz. cheddar cheese, grated
- 4oz. black olives, pitted and diced
- Salt and black pepper- to taste
- 15oz. canned tomatillos, diced

Directions:

1. Start by throwing all the Ingredients into the Slow cooker and mix them well.

2. Cover it and cook for 5 6 hours on Low Settings.

3. Shred the slow-cooked chicken and return to the pot.

4. Mix well and garnish as desired.

5. Serve warm.

Nutrition: Calories 427 Fat 31.1 g Carbs 5 g Sugar 12.4 g Fiber 19.8 g Protein 23.5 g

DINNER

18. Cod & Peas With Sour Cream

Preparation Time: 6 minutes

Cooking time: 1 hrs.

Servings: 6

Ingredients

- 1 tablespoon of fresh parsley
- 1 garlic clove, diced
- 1/2 lb.. froz.en peas
- 1/2 teaspoon of paprika
- 1 cup of sour cream
- 1/2 cup of white wine

Directions:

1. Start by throwing all the Ingredients: into your Slow cooker except sour cream.
2. Cover its lid and cook for 1 hour on High setting.
3. Once done, remove its lid and give it a stir.
4. Stir in sour cream and mix it gently

5. Serve warm.

Nutrition: Calories 349 Fat 31.9 g Sodium 237 mg Carbs 1.6 g Sugar 1.4 g Fiber 3.4 g Protein 11 g

19. Slow Cooker Tuna Steaks

Preparation Time: 6 minutes Cooking time: 4 hrs.

Servings: 6

Ingredients

- 4 tuna steaks
- 3 garlic cloves, crushed
- 1 lemon, sliced into 8 slices
- 1/2 cup white wine

Directions:

1. Reduce the white wine in a pot by simmering until the strong alcoholic smell is cooked off.
2. Rub the tuna steaks with olive oil, and sprinkle with salt and pepper.
3. Place the tuna steaks into the Slow Cooker.
4. Sprinkle the crushed garlic on top of the tuna steaks.
5. Place 2 lemon slices on top of each tuna steak.
6. Pour the reduced wine into the pot.
7. Secure the lid onto the pot and set the temperature to HIGH.
8. Cook for 3 hours. Serve with a drizzle of leftover liquid from the pot, and a side of crispy greens!

Nutrition: Calories 123 Fat 21 g Sodium 213 mg Carbs 2 g Sugar 2 g Fiber 3g Protein 15 g

20. Tilapia And Radish Bites

Preparation Time: 5 minutes

Cooking time: 2 hrs.

Servings: 2

Ingredients

- 1 1/2 cups radishes, halved
- 1 teaspoon sweet paprika
- 1/2 teaspoon dried rosemary
- 1/4 teaspoon ground black pepper
- 1/2 teaspoon salt
- 9 oz. tilapia fillet, boneless and cubed
- 2 oz. Cheddar cheese, sliced
- 1/4 cup veggie stock

Directions:

1. In the slow cooker, mix the radishes with the fish and the other ingredients and toss.
2. Close the lid and cook the fish for 5 hours on High.

Nutrition: Calories 251, Fat 8.4, Fiber 0.2, Carbs 1.3, Protein 6.6

21. Shrimp & Pepper Stew

Preparation Time: 5 minutes

Cooking time: 2 hrs.

Servings: 4

Ingredients

- 14 oz.. canned diced tomatoes
- 1/4 cup of yellow onion, peeled and diced
- 2 tablespoon of lime juice
- 1/4 cup of olive oil
- 11/2 lb.s. shrimp, peeled and deveined
- 1/4 cup of red pepper, roasted and diced
- 1 garlic clove, peeled and diced
- 1 cup of coconut milk
- 1/4 cup of fresh cilantro, diced
- Salt and black pepper ground, to taste

Directions:

1. Start by throwing all the Ingredients: into your Slow cooker except shrimp.
2. Cover its lid and cook for 2 hours on Low setting.
3. Once done, remove its lid and give it a stir.

4. Stir in shrimp and continue cooking for 1 hour on low heat.

5. Serve warm.

Nutrition: Calories 392 Fat 40.4 g Sodium 423 mg Carbs 2.7 g Sugar 3 g Protein 21 g

22. Seafood Stew

Preparation Time: 5 minutes

Cooking time: 4 hrs.

Servings: 4

Ingredients

- Haddock fillets – 1/2 lb.., cut into 1-inch pieces
- Raw shrimp – 1/2 lb.., peeled, deveined
- Lump crab meat – 1/2 (6 oz..) can, drained
- Chopped clams – 1/2 (6 oz..) can, with its liquid
- Clam juice – 4 oz..
- Olive oil – 1/2 tbsp..
- Medium onion – 1, chopped
- Garlic – 3 cloves, minced
- Celery – 2 ribs, chopped
- Tomato paste – 1/2 (6 oz..) can
- Diced tomatoes – 1/2 (28 oz..) can, with liquid
- White wine – 1/4 cup
- Red wine vinegar – 1/2 tbsp..
- Italian seasoning – 1 tsp.
- Bay leaf – 1

- Erythritol – 1/4 tsp.
- Parsley – 2 tbsp.. chopped
- Salt to taste

Directions:

1. Except for seafood and parsley, add all the ingredients to the Crock-Pot.
2. Cover and cook on low for 3 to 4 hours.
3. Add the seafood and mix well.
4. Cover and cook on high for 30 minutes. Stir a couple of times while it is cooking.
5. Discard the bay leaf. Add parsley.
6. Mix well and serve.

Nutrition: Calories: 201 Fat: 4g Carbs: 1.8g Protein: 30.4g

23. Creamy Seafood Chowder

Preparation Time: 5 minutes Cooking time: 5 hrs.

Servings: 6

Ingredients

- Garlic – 5 cloves, crushed
- Small onion – 1, finely chopped
- Prawns – 1 cup
- Shrimp – 1 cup
- Whitefish – 1 cup
- Full-fat cream – 2 cups
- Dry white wine – 1 cup
- A handful of fresh parsley, finely chopped
- Olive oil – 2 tbsp..

Directions:

1. Drizzle oil into the Crock-Pot.
2. Add the white fish, shrimp, prawns, onion, garlic, cream, wine, salt, and pepper into the pot. Stir to mix.
3. Cover with the lid and cook on low for 5 hours.
4. Sprinkle with fresh parsley and serve.

Nutrition: Calories: 225 Fat: 9.6g Carbs: 5.g Protein: 21.4g

24. Salmon Cake

Preparation Time: 5 minutes

Cooking time: 4 hrs.

Servings: 4

Ingredients

- Eggs – 4, lightly beaten
- Heavy cream – 3 tbsp..
- Baby spinach – 1 cup, roughly chopped
- Smoked salmon strips – 4 ounces, chopped
- A handful of fresh coriander, roughly chopped
- Olive oil – 2 tbsp..
- Salt and pepper to taste

Directions:

1. Drizzle oil into the Crock-Pot.
2. Place the spinach, cream, beaten egg, salmon, salt, and pepper into the pot and mix to combine.
3. Cover with the lid and cook on low for 4 hours.
4. Sprinkle with fresh coriander and serve.

Nutrition: Calories: 277 Fat: 20.8g Carbs: 1.1g Protein: 22.5g

25. Lemon-Butter Fish

Preparation Time: 5 minutes

Cooking time: 5 hrs.

Servings: 4

Ingredients

- Fresh white fish – 4 fillets
- Butter - 1 1/2 ounce, soft but not melted
- Garlic cloves – 2, crushed
- Lemon – 1 (juice and zest)
- A handful of fresh parsley, finely chopped
- Salt and pepper to taste
- Olive oil – 2 tbsp..

Directions:

1. Combine the butter, garlic, zest of one lemon, and chopped parsley to a bowl.
2. Drizzle oil into the Crock-Pot.
3. Season the fish with salt and pepper and place into the pot.
4. Place a dollop of lemon butter onto each fish fillet and gently spread it out.
5. Cover with the lid and cook on low for 5 hours.

6. Serve each fish fillet with a generous spoonful of melted lemon butter from the bottom of the pot. Drizzle with lemon juice and serve.

Nutrition: Calories: 202 Fat: 13.4g Carbs: 1.3g Protein: 20.3g

26. Salmon with Green Beans

Preparation Time: 5 minutes

Cooking time: 3 hrs.

Servings: 4

Ingredients

- Salmon fillets – 4, skin on
- Garlic – 4 cloves, crushed
- Broccoli – 1/2 head, cut into florets
- Froz.en green beans – 2 cups
- Olive oil – 3 tbsp.., divided
- Salt and pepper to taste
- Water – 1/4 cup

Directions:

1. Add the olive oil into the Crock-Pot.
2. Season the salmon with salt and pepper and place into the pot (skin-side down). Add the water.
3. Place garlic, beans, and broccoli on top of the salmon. Season with salt and pepper.
4. Drizzle some more oil over the veggies and fish.
5. Cover with the lid and cook on high for 3 hours.

6. Serve.

Nutrition: Calories: 278 Fat: 17.8g Carbs: 1g Protein: 24.5g

27. Coconut Fish Curry

Preparation Time: 5 minutes

Cooking time: 4 hrs.

Servings: 4

Ingredients

- Large white fish fillets – 4, cut into chunks
- Garlic cloves – 4, crushed
- Small onion – 1, finely chopped
- Ground turmeric – 1 tsp.
- Yellow curry paste – 2 tbsp..
- Fish stock – 2 cups
- Full-fat coconut milk – 2 cans
- Lime – 1
- Fresh coriander as needed, roughly chopped
- Olive oil – 2 tbsp..
- Salt and pepper to taste

Directions:

1. Add olive oil into the Crock-Pot.
2. Add the coconut milk, stock, fish, curry paste, turmeric, onion, garlic, salt, and pepper to the pot. Stir to combine.

3. Cover with the lid and cook on high for 4 hours.
4. Drizzle with lime juice and fresh coriander and serve.

Nutrition: Calories: 562 Fat: 49.9g Carbs: 1.3g Protein: 20.6g

28. Coconut Lime Mussels

Preparation Time: 5 minutes

Cooking time: 2 hrs.

Servings: 4

Ingredients

- Fresh mussels – 16
- Garlic – 4 cloves
- Full-fat coconut milk – 1 1/2 cups
- Red chili – 1/2, finely chopped
- Lime – 1, juiced
- Fish stock – 1/2 cup
- A handful of fresh coriander
- Olive oil – 2 tbsp..
- Salt and pepper to taste

Directions:

1. Add olive oil into the Crock-Pot.
2. Add the coconut milk, garlic, chili, fish stock, salt, pepper, and juice of one lime to the pot. Stir to mix.
3. Cover with the lid and cook on high for 2 hours.
4. Remove the lid, place mussels into the liquid, and cover with the lid.

5. Cook until mussels open, about 20 minutes.

6. Serve the mussels with pot sauce. Garnish with fresh coriander.

Nutrition: Calories: 342 Fat: 30.2g Carbs: 1.3g Protein: 10.9g

29. Calamari, Prawn, and Shrimp Pasta Sauce

Preparation Time: 5 minutes

Cooking time: 3 hrs.

Servings: 6

Ingredients

- Calamari – 1 cup
- Prawns – 1 cup
- Shrimp – 1 cup
- Garlic – 6 cloves, crushed
- Tomatoes – 4, chopped
- Dried mixed herbs – 1 tsp.
- Balsamic vinegar - 1 tbsp..
- Olive oil – 2 tbsp..
- Salt and pepper to taste
- Water – 1/2 cup

Directions:

1. Add oil into the Crock-Pot.
2. Add the tomatoes, garlic, shrimp, prawns, calamari, mixed herbs, balsamic vinegar, water, salt, and pepper. Stir to mix.
3. Cover with the lid and cook on high for 3 hours.

4. Serve with zucchini noodles or veggies.

Nutrition: Calories: 372 Fat: 14.6g Carbs: 5g Protein: 55.1g

30. Cabbage Stew

Preparation time: 15 minutes

Cooking time: 3 Hours

Servings: 2

Ingredients

- cups white cabbage, shredded
- ½ cup tomato juice
- 1 teaspoon ground white pepper
- 1 cup cauliflower, chopped
- ½ cup potato, chopped
- 1 cup of water

Directions:

1 Put cabbage, potato, and cauliflower in the Slow Cooker.

2 Add tomato juice, ground white pepper, and water. Stir the stew Ingredients: and close the lid.

3 Cook the stew on high for hours.

Nutrition: 57 calories, 2.8g protein, 13.3g carbohydrates, 0.2g fat, 3.9g fiber, 0mg cholesterol, 196mg sodium, 503mg potassium.

31. Sweet Potato & Sausage Soup

Preparation time: 15 minutes

Cooking time: 7 Hours And 35 Minutes

Servings: 6 (12.4 Ounces per Serving)

Ingredients

- 1 lb. sausage links, pork or chicken
- large sweet potatoes, cubed
- 1 onion, chopped
- 1 glass red wine
- tablespoons tomato sauce
- Olive oil
- cups water
- Salt and pepper to taste and other seasonings
- 1 cup of bacon, cooked, cubed
- 1 cup smoked ham, cooked, cubed
- 1 red pepper, diced

Directions:

1 Chop the onion into cubes. Grease a frying pan and sauté onion until golden in color, for about six minutes.

2 Add the cubed ham and bacon. Add cubed potatoes and salt and pepper to taste.

3 Pour in wine and stir. Place all Ingredients: in Slow Cooker.

4 Add the water and cover and cook on LOW for 6-7 hours.

5 Add the chopped pepper and tomato sauce and cook on LOW for an additional 30 minutes more.

6 Serve hot.

Nutrition: Calories: 126.71, Total Fat: 2.02 g, Saturated Fat: 0.99 g, Cholesterol: 18.33 mg, Sodium: 787.22 mg, Potassium: 215.12 mg, Total Carbohydrates: 6.95 g, Fiber: 0.52 g, Sugar: 1.26 g, Protein: 15.3 g

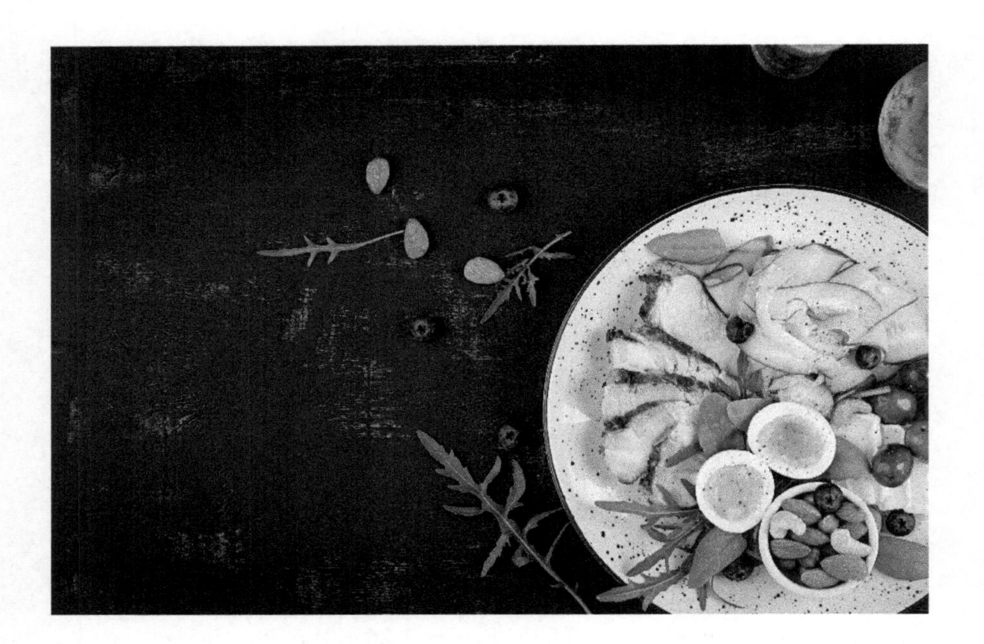

MEAT RECIPES

32. Root Beer Pulled Pork Sandwich

Preparation time: 10 minutes

Cooking time: 7 hours

Servings: 4

Ingredients:

- 1-2 cans root beer soda
- cups BBQ sauce, plus some more for serving
- pork loins, about 1 – 1 ½ pounds
- Salt and Pepper
- ½ cup prepared slaw
- rolls

Directions:

1 Season the pork loins with pepper and salt.

2 Place pork in slow cooker, and pour enough root beer and BBQ sauce to almost cover it.

3 Cook on LOW for 7-8 hours.

4 Remove pork and discard liquid.

5 Shred the pork.

6 To serve, warm the sandwich rolls. Add shredded pork with some barbecue sauce. Top with slaw.

7 Serve warm.

Nutrition: calories 446, fat 18, carbs 45, protein 21

POULTRY

33. Slow cooker Chicken Adobo

Preparation Time: 10 minutes

Cooking Time: 8 hours

Servings: 6

Ingredients:

- 1/4 cup of apple cider vinegar
- 12 chicken drumsticks
- 1 onion, diced into slices
- 2 tablespoons of olive oil
- 10 cloves garlic, smashed
- 1 cup of gluten-free tamari
- 1/4 cup of diced green onion

Directions:

1. Place the drumsticks in the Slow cooker and then add the remaining ingredients on top.
2. Cover it and cook for 8 hours on Low Settings.
3. Mix gently, then serve warm.

Nutrition: Calories 249 Total Fat 11.9 g Saturated Fat 1.7 g Cholesterol 78 mg Total Carbs 1.8 g Fiber 1.1 g Sugar 0.3 g Sodium 79 mg Potassium 131 mg Protein 25 g

SIDE DISH RECIPES

34. Broccoli Mix

Preparation time: 15 minutes

Cooking time: 2 Hours

Servings: 10

Ingredients

- `6 cups broccoli florets
- `1 and ½ cups cheddar cheese, shredded
- `10 ounces canned cream of celery soup
- `½ teaspoon Worcestershire sauce
- `¼ cup yellow onion, chopped
- `Salt and black pepper to the taste
- `1 cup crackers, crushed
- `2 tablespoons soft butter

Directions:

1. In a bowl, mix broccoli with cream of celery soup, cheese, salt, pepper, onion and Worcestershire sauce, toss and transfer to your Slow cooker.

2. Add butter, toss again, sprinkle crackers, cover and cook on High for hours.
3. Serve as a side dish.

Nutrition: calories 159, fat 11, fiber 1, carbs 11, protein 6

35. Roasted Beets

Preparation time: 15 minutes

Cooking time: 4 Hours

Servings: 5

Ingredients

- `10 small beets
- `5 teaspoons olive oil
- `A pinch of salt and black pepper

Directions:

1. Divide each beet on a tin foil piece, drizzle oil, season them with salt and pepper, rub well, wrap beets, place them in your Slow cooker, cover and cook on High for 4 hours.
2. Unwrap beets, cool them down a bit, peel, and slice and serve them as a side dish.

Nutrition: calories 100, fat 2, fiber 2, carbs 4, protein 5

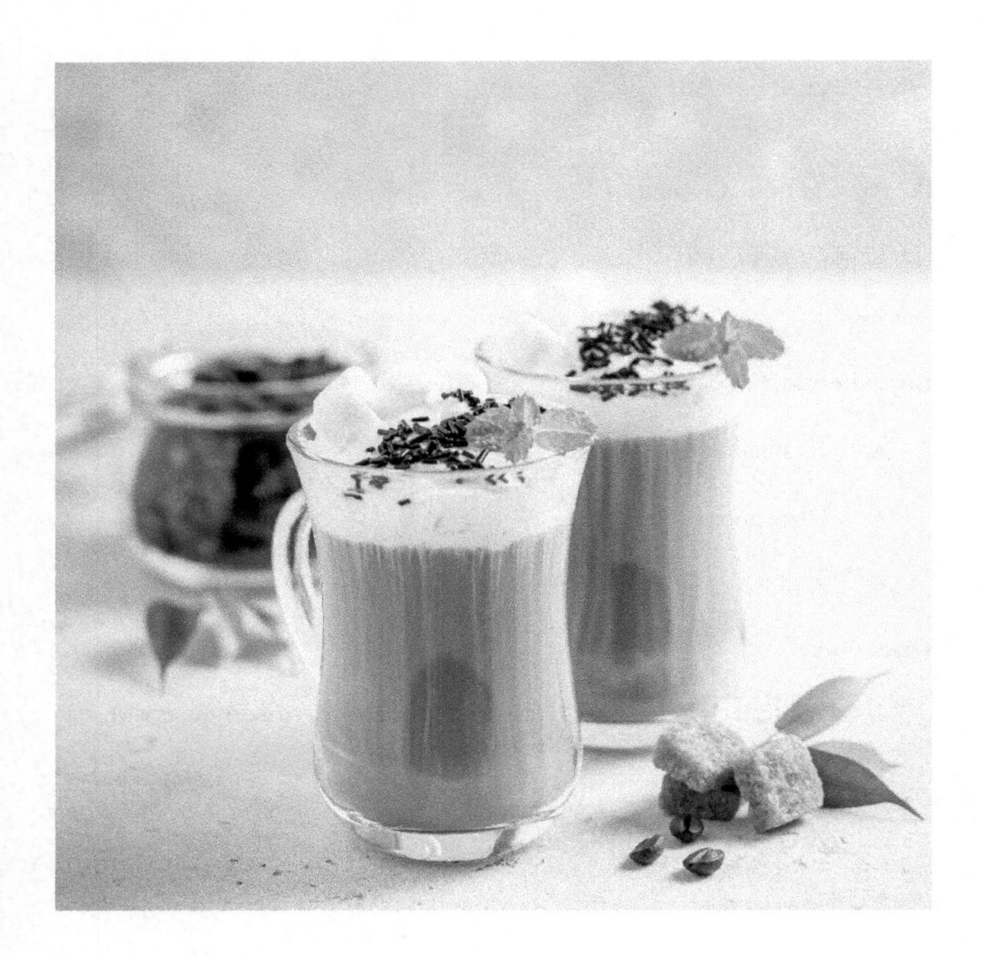

VEGETABLES

36. Coconut Flour"Porridge" With Blueberries and Cinnamon

Difficulty: Easy

Preparation time: 40 minutes

Cooking time: 2 ½ hours

Servings: 4

Ingredients

- `⅔ cups of coconut flour
- `⅓ cup flaxseed flour
- `⅔ cup unsweetened, coconut cream
- `1 tbsp. of ghee
- `1 tsp of agave syrup
- `1 tbsp. of blueberries
- `1 tsp of cinnamon

Directions:

1. Place all the first four Ingredients together in the slow cooker to make a thick paste.

2. Set to cook on low heat for 2 ½ hours to make a thick, creamy porridge.
3. Transfer onto a big bowl (or two smaller bowls) and drizzle with a bit of agave syrup. Add the cinnamon and blueberries on top.

Nutrition: Calories: 453, Fat: 39g, Carbs: 12g, Protein: 14g.

37. Squash Noodles

Preparation time: 15 minutes

Cooking time: 4 hours

Servings: 4

Ingredients:

- `1-pound butternut squash, seeded, halved
- `1 tablespoon vegan butter
- `1 teaspoon salt
- `½ teaspoon garlic powder
- `1 cups of water

Directions

1. Pour water in the slow cooker.
2. Add butternut squash and close the lid.
3. Cook the vegetable on high for 4 hours.
4. Then drain water and shred the squash flesh with the fork's help and transfer in the bowl.
5. Add garlic powder, salt, and butter. Mix the squash noodles.

Nutrition 78 calories, 1.2g Protein, 13.5g carbohydrates, 3g fat, 2.3g fiber, 8mg cholesterol, 612mg sodium, 406mg potassium

38. Thyme Tomatoes

Preparation time: 10 minutes

Cooking time: 5 hours

Servings: 4

Ingredients:

- `1-pound tomatoes, sliced
- `1 tablespoon dried thyme
- `1 teaspoon salt
- `1 tablespoons olive oil
- `1 tablespoon apple cider vinegar
- `½ cup of water

Directions

1. Place ingredients in the slow cooker and close the lid.
2. Cook the tomatoes on Low for 5 hours.

Nutrition 83 calories, 1.1g Protein, 4.9g carbohydrates, 7.3g fat, 1.6g fiber, 0mg cholesterol, 588mg sodium, 277mg potassium

39. Quinoa Dolma

Preparation time: 15 minutes

Cooking time: 3 hours

Servings: 6

Ingredients:

- `sweet peppers, seeded
- `1 cup quinoa, cooked
- `½ cup corn kernels, cooked
- `1 teaspoon chili flakes
- `1 cup of water
- `½ cup tomato juice

Directions

1. Mix quinoa with corn kernels, and chili flakes.
2. Fill the sweet peppers with quinoa mixture and put in the slow cooker.
3. Add water and tomato juice.
4. Close the lid and cook the peppers on High for 3 hours.

Nutrition 171 calories, 6.6g Protein, 33.7g carbohydrates, 2.3g fat, 4.8g fiber, 0mg cholesterol, 29mg sodium, 641mg potassium

40. Creamy Puree

Preparation time: 10 minutes

Cooking time: 4 hours

Servings: 4

Ingredients:

- `1 cups potatoes, chopped
- `1 cups of water
- `1 tablespoon vegan butter
- `¼ cup cream
- `1 teaspoon salt

Directions

1. Pour water in the slow cooker.
2. Add potatoes and salt.
3. Cook the vegetables on high for 4 hours.
4. Then drain water, add butter, and cream.
5. Mash the potatoes until smooth.

Nutrition 87 calories, 1.4g Protein, 12.3g carbohydrates, 3.8g fat, 1.8g fiber, 10mg cholesterol, 617mg sodium, 314mg potassium

FISH & SEAFOOD

41. Shrimp and Salmon Skewers

Preparation Time: 10 minutes

Cooking time: 2 hours

Servings: 4

Ingredients:

- `9 oz shrimps, peeled
- `9 ounces salmon fillets, boneless and cubed
- `1 teaspoon garlic powder
- `1 teaspoon ginger powder
- `1 tablespoon lime juice
- `1/3 teaspoon oregano, dried
- `1 tablespoon sesame oil
- `1 teaspoon heavy cream
- `¾ cup of water

Directions:

1 String the shrimps and salmon into the skewers one-by-one.

2 After this, pour water into the slow cooker.

3 Arrange the shrimp and salmon skewers in the slow cooker, and add the rest of the ingredients as well.

4 Close the lid and cook shrimps for 1.5 hours on High.

5 Then transfer the cooked shrimp skewers to the plates and sprinkle with slow cooker gravy.

Nutrition: calories 185, fat 5, carbs 5, protein 14

APPETIZERS & SNACKS

42. Sweet Coconut Cassava

Preparation Time: 15 Minutes

Cooking Time: 1 hour

Servings: 4

Ingredients:

- 2lb.s. yellow cassava, chopped into large chunks
- 1cup white sugar
- 1can thick coconut cream
- 1/4tsp.. coconut oil
- 4cups water
- 1/8tsp.. vanilla extract
- Pinch of salt

Directions:

1 Lightly grease the insides of the Instant Pot Pressure Cooker with coconut oil.

2 Pour water. Add in yellow cassava, sugar, and salt.

3 Lock the lid in place. Press the high pressure and cook for 7 minutes.

4 When the beep sounds, Choose the Quick Pressure Release. This will depressurize for 7 minutes. Remove the lid.

5 Tip in coconut cream and vanilla extract. Allow residual heat cook the last two ingredients. Adjust seasoning according to your preferred taste.

6 To serve, ladle equal amounts into dessert bowls.

Nutrition: Calories 345 Fat 12 Fiber 9 Carbs 2.9 Protein 29

43. Tofu With Salted Caramel Pearls

Preparation Time: 5 Minutes

Cooking Time: 1 hour

Servings: 4

Ingredients:

- 1cup tapioca pearls, no need to soak
- 2packs 12 oz.. soft silken tofu
- 5cups water, divided
- 1cup brown sugar
- 1/16tsp.. salt

Directions:

1 Pour tapioca pearls and water into the Instant Pot Pressure Cooker slow cooker.

2 Lock the lid in place. Press the high pressure and cook for 10 minutes.

3 When the beep sounds, Choose Natural Pressure Release. Depressurizing would take 20 minutes. Remove the lid.

4 Reposition the lid and cook for another 5 minutes on high.

5 When the beep sounds, Choose Natural Pressure Release. Depressurizing would take 20 minutes. Remove the lid. Pour out contents of the pressure cooker over colander to drain.

6 Press the "saute" button. Put back tapioca pearls to the slow cooker. Add silken tofu, brown sugar, and salt.

7 Cook for 10 minutes or until the caramel thickens. Turn off the machine.

8 Meanwhile, scoop silken tofu into heat-resistant cups. Pour tapioca pearls and caramel on top. Serve.

Nutrition: Calories 125 Fat 18 Fiber 19 Carbs 1 Protein 13

44. Homemade HUMMUS

Preparation Time: 5 Minutes

Cooking Time: 1 hour

Servings: 4

Ingredients:

- 6cups water
- 1cup dry chickpeas
- 2fresh bay leaves
- 4garlic cloves, peeled
- 5pieces crackers per person as base
- 3Tbsp.. tahini
- 1/4tsp.. cumin powder
- 1/2cup lemon juice, freshly squeezed
- 1/4tsp.. salt
- 1/16tsp.. toasted black sesame seeds
- 1/16tsp.. toasted white sesame seeds
- 1/16tsp.. red pepper flakes
- 2Tbsp.. extra virgin olive oil
- 1sprig of basil

Directions:

1 Place chickpeas, bay leaves, garlic cloves, and water into the Instant Pot Pressure Cooker.

2 Lock the lid in place. Press the high pressure and cook for 20 minutes.

3 When the beep sounds, Choose Natural Pressure Release. Depressurizing would take 20 minutes. Remove the lid. Reserve 1 cup of cooking liquid. Discard the rest.

4 Transfer chickpeas to an immersion blender, along with the cooking liquid. Season with tahini, cumin powder, lemon juice, and salt. Process until smooth. Adjust seasoning according to your preferred taste.

5 Pour chickpeas into a bowl. Garnish with toasted black and white sesame seeds, red pepper flakes, basil, and olive oil. Serve with crackers.

6 Store leftovers in the fridge. Use as needed.

Nutrition: Calories 122 Fat 11 Fiber 21 Carbs 1.3 Protein 13

45. Corn Coconut Pudding

Preparation Time: 5 Minutes

Cooking Time: 45 minutes

Servings: 3

Ingredients:

- 3cups water
- 1cup corn kernels
- 1/2cup sticky rice
- 1/4cup ripe jackfruit, shredded,
- 1/4tsp.. vanilla extract
- 1/2cup sugar
- 1/8tsp.. nutmeg powder
- 1/16tsp.. salt
- 2cans thick coconut cream, divided

Directions:

1 Pour water, sticky rice, jackfruit, corn kernels, 1 can of coconut cream, nutmeg powder, vanilla extract, white sugar, and salt in the Instant Pot Pressure Cooker.

2 Lock the lid in place. Press the high pressure and cook for 7 minutes.

3 When the beep sounds, Choose the Quick Pressure Release. This will depressurize for 7 minutes. Remove the lid.

4 Tip in the remaining can of coconut cream. Allow residual heat cook the coconut cream. Adjust seasoning according to your preferred taste.

5 To serve, ladle equal amounts into dessert bowls.

Nutrition: Calories 213 Fat 12 Fiber 21 Carbs 2 Protein 13

DESSERT

46. Brownie with Cherries

Preparation Time: 30 minutes

Cooking Time 50 minutes

Servings: 4

Ingredients:

- `200 g chocolate
- `200 g butter
- `4 eggs
- `200 g sugar
- `100 g flour
- `1 glass morello cherries
- `1 tbsp.. potato starch
- `1 pinch cinnamon
- `1 tsp.. sugar
- `Butter for the mold

Directions:

1. Preheat the oven to 210 C. Grease a baking pan 24 cm in diameter.

2. Melt the chocolate over a hot water bath, take it off the stove and stir in the cold butter little by little. Stir the mixture until creamy. Separate the eggs. Beat the egg white until stiff, then beat the egg yolks with the sugar until frothy until the mixture turns white and creamy. Carefully stir into the cooled chocolate and butter mixture. Fold in the egg whites. Sift the flour over it and fold it carefully. Put the dough in the greased baking pan and place on the middle rack for 20 minutes
3. For the cherry sauce, put the cherries and the liquid (except for 3 tablespoons) in a saucepan, heat with sugar. Put the cinnamon, starch, and the 3 tablespoons of juice in a cup and stir until smooth. Add the mixed starch to the cherries while stirring, bring to the boil, and set aside.
4. Cut the cake into 15 squares and then into triangles. Arrange two triangles with the cherry sauce on plates and serve.

Nutrition: Calories 321 Fat 19 Fiber 3 Carbs 1.9 Protein 21

47. Coffee-Chocolate Cake

Preparation Time: 30 minutes

Cooking Time 50 minutes

Servings: 6

Ingredients:

- `150 g dark chocolate 70% cocoa content
- `100 g milk chocolate with 30% cocoa content
- `100 g soft butter
- `2 tsp.. crème fraîche at least 30% fat
- `100 g almond kernels
- `3 eggs
- `200 g brown sugar
- `1/2 tsp.. salt 180 g flour
- `10 g cocoa powder
- `10 g baking powder
- `1 tbsp.. rum
- `20 g instant coffee

Directions:

1. Chop both kinds of chocolate roughly and melt it over a hot water bath together with butter. Slowly cool, and then stir in the fresh

cream. To 180 C Preheat oven. Line a parchment paper baking sheet. Cut the almonds very hard. In a bowl, add the sugar and salt to the eggs until the sugar is dissolved. Mix in the chocolate-butter blend gradually. Stir. Mix the meal and the baked powder with the cocoa and sieve. Warm down the rum, dissolve the coffee in it and add the meal and almonds to the dough. Place and smooth the dough on the baker. Bake brownies for 35-40 minutes in a hot oven on the center rack (test the stick!). Allow the brownies to cool down and chop (about.

2. Wash the orange with hot water for garnishing, rub it dry and remove the peel with fine zest. Half the fruit, squeeze the juice, and then enter into a small cup of sugar. Additionally, add sugar and reduce to syrup the mixture. Add the orange zest and allow it to dry until the syrup has a golden brown color.

Nutrition: Calories 187 Fat 11 Fiber 3 Carbs 2.5 Protein 12

48. Brownies with Coffee

Preparation Time: 15 minutes

Cooking Time 50 minutes

Servings: 6-8

Ingredients:

- `350 g dark coverture
- `200 g chopped walnut kernels
- `6 eggs
- `300 g sugar
- `Scraped pulp of a vanilla pod
- `1 pinch salt
- `200 ml oil
- `150 g flour
- `3 tbsp.. cocoa powder
- `2 tsp.. baking powder
- `100 ml espresso
- `Powdered sugar

Directions:

1. Coarsely chop 100 g coverture. Crush the remaining coverture and melt it in a bowl in a hot water bath. Mix eggs with sugar, vanilla pulp, and salt until frothy. Add oil and stir briefly until smooth.
2. Mix the flour, cocoa, and baking powder and fold carefully into the batter. Finally, fold the melted coverture, chopped walnuts, and chopped coverture with half of the espresso into the batter.
3. Place the dough on a baking sheet (30 x 20 cm) lined with baking paper and smooth it out. Bake in the preheated oven (180 top and bottom heat, middle rack) for about 30 minutes.
4. Take out and let cool slightly. Then spread the rest of the espresso on the still-warm cake and let it cool down. Cut into pieces for serving and dust with powdered sugar.

Nutrition: Calories 213 Fat 21 Fiber 5 Carbs 2.5 Protein 11

49. Sauerkraut brownies with blackberries

Preparation Time: 25 minutes

Cooking Time 1 hour

Servings: 6-8

Ingredients:

- `100 g warm butter
- `120 g coconut blossom sugar
- `1 vanilla pod
- `200 g spelled flour
- `1 packet baking powder
- `100 g cocoa powder
- `1 pinch salt
- `3 eggs
- `300 ml milk
- `160 g wine sauerkraut
- `125 g blackberry
- `4 tbsp.. almond sticks

Directions:

1. Beat the blossom sugar butter and cocoa until it is creamy. Scrape out the pulp and half the vanilla put along with the pulp. Flour, baking powder, cocoa, salt, eggs, and milk in a whisk of vanilla pulp.
2. Rinse the sauerkraut in hot water, thoroughly squeeze out and cut into tiny parts. Remove the mixture of the coconut butter and almond sticks into the batter.
3. Wash the blackberries and drain them. In a baking platter with baked paper, press the blackberries and bake for 30 to 35 minutes (stick test), in a preheated fire oven at 180 C.
4. Cool and serve the brownie sauerkraut and blackberries.

Nutrition: Calories 154 Fat 21 Fiber 11 Carbs: 4.3 Protein 11

50. Delicious Apple Crisp

Preparation Time: 10 minutes

Cooking Time: 3 hours

Servings: 8

Ingredients:

- 2lb.s apples, peeled & sliced
- 1/2 cup butter
- 1/4 tsp. ground nutmeg
- 1/2 tsp. ground cinnamon
- 2/3 cup brown sugar
- 2/3 cup flour
- 2/3 cup old-fashioned oats

Directions:

1. Add sliced apples into the cooking pot.
2. In a mixing bowl, mix together flour, nutmeg, cinnamon, sugar, and oats.
3. Add butter into the flour mixture and mix until the mixture is crumbly.
4. Sprinkle flour mixture over sliced apples.
5. Cover instant pot aura with lid.

6. Select slow cook mode and cook on HIGH for 2-3 hours.

7. Top with vanilla ice-cream and serve.

Nutrition: Calories 251 Fat 12, Carbs 3.3, Protein 2.1 g

30 DAY MEAL PLAN

DAY	BREAKFAST	LUNCH	DINNER	DESSERTS
1	Egg Sausage Breakfast Casserole	Garlic Duck Breast	Pork Chops	Chocolate Mousse
2	Vegetable Omelet	Thyme Lamb Chops	Spicy Pork & Spinach Stew	Chocolate Chia Pudding With Almonds
3	Cheese Bacon Quiche	Autumn Pork Stew	Stuffed Taco Peppers	Coconut Macadamia Chia Pudding
4	Egg Breakfast Casserole	Handmade Sausage Stew	Chinese Pulled Pork	Keto Chocolate Mug
5	Cauliflower Breakfast Casserole	Marinated Beef Tenderloin	Bacon Wrapped Pork Loin	Vanilla Chia Pudding
6	Veggie Frittata	Chicken Liver Sauté	Lamb Barbacoa	Choco Lava Cake
7	Feta Spinach Quiche	Chicken In Bacon	Balsamic Pork Tenderloin	Coconut Cup Cakes
8	Cauliflower Mashed	Whole Chicken	Spicy Pork	Easy Chocolate Cheesecake
9	Kalua Pork With Cabbage	Duck Rolls	Zesty Garlic Pulled Pork	Chocolate Chip Brownie
10	Creamy Pork	Keto Adobo	Ranch	Coconut

	Chops	Chicken	Pork Chops	Cookies
11	Beef Taco Filling	Cayenne Pepper Drumsticks	Pork Chile Verde	Choco Pie
12	Flavorful Steak Fajitas	Keto Bbq Chicken Wings	Ham Soup	Keto Blueberry Muffins
13	Garlic Herb Pork	Sweet Corn Pilaf	Beef And Broccoli	Keto Oven-Baked Brie Cheese
14	Garlic Thyme Lamb Chops	Mediterranean Vegetable Mix	Korean Barbecue Beef	Keto Vanilla Pound Cake
15	Pork Tenderloin	Spaghetti Cottage Cheese Casserole	Garlic Chicken	Almond Roll With Pumpkin Cream Cheese Filling
16	Smoky Pork With Cabbage	Meatballs With Coconut Gravy	Lamb Shanks	No Bake Low Carb Lemon Strawberry Cheesecake
17	Italian Frittata	Fresh Dal	Jamaican Jerk Pork Roast	Pecan Cheesecake
18	Easy Mexican Chicken	Pulled Pork Salad	Salmon	Blueberry And Zucchini Muffins
19	Cherry Tomatoes Thyme	Garlic Pork Belly	Coconut Chicken	Coffee Mousse

	Asparagus Frittata			
20	Healthy Veggie Omelet	Sesame Seed Shrimp	Mahi Mahi Taco Wraps	Chocolate Cake
21	Scrambled Eggs With Smoked Salmon	Chicken Liver Pate	Shrimp Tacos	Sweet Potato Brownies
22	Persian Omelet Slow cooker	Cod Fillet In Coconut Flakes	Fish Curry	Raspberry Brownies
23	Keto Slow cooker Tasty Onions	Prawn Stew	Salmon With Creamy Lemon Sauce	Brownie Cheesecake
24	Crustless Slow cooker Spinach Quiche	Pork-Jalapeno Bowl	Salmon With Lemon-Caper Sauce	Zucchini-Brownies
25	Eggplant Pate With Breadcrumbs	Chicken Marsala	Spicy Barbecue Shrimp	Bean Brownies
26	Red Beans With The Sweet Peas	Chickpeas Soup	Lemon Dill Halibut	Luscious Walnut Chocolate Brownies
27	Nutritious Burrito Bowl	Hot And Delicious Soup	Coconut Cilantro Curry Shrimp	Gluten-Free Chocolate Cake
28	Quinoa Curry	Delicious	Shrimp In	Brownies

		Eggplant Salad	Marinara Sauce	With Nuts
29	Ham Pitta Pockets	Tasty Black Beans Soup	Garlic Shrimp	Halloween Brownies
30	Breakfast Meatloaf	Rich Sweet Potato Soup	Lemon Pepper Tilapia	Raw Brownies With Cashew Nuts

CONVERSION TABLES

Volume Equivalents (Liquid)

US STANDARD	US STANDARD (OUNCES)	METRIC (APPROXIMATE)
2 tablespoons	1 fl. oz...	30 mL
1/4 cup	2 fl. oz...	60 mL
1/2 cup	4 fl. oz...	120 mL
1 cup	8 fl. oz...	240 mL
11/2 cups	12 fl. oz...	355 mL
2 cups or 1 pint	16 fl. oz...	475 mL
4 cups or 1 quart	32 fl. oz...	1 L
1 gallon	128 fl. oz...	4 L

Volume Equivalents (Dry)

US STANDARD	METRIC (APPROXIMATE)
1/4 teaspoon	1 mL
1/2 teaspoon	2 mL
1 teaspoon	5 mL
1 tablespoon	15 mL
1/4 cup	59 mL
cup	79 mL
1/2 cup	118 mL
1 cup	177 mL

Oven Temperatures

FAHRENHEIT (F)	CELSIUS (C) (APPROXIMATE)
250°F	120 °C
300°F	150°C
325°F	165°C
350°F	180°C
375°F	190°C
400°F	200°C
425°F	220°C
450°F	230°C

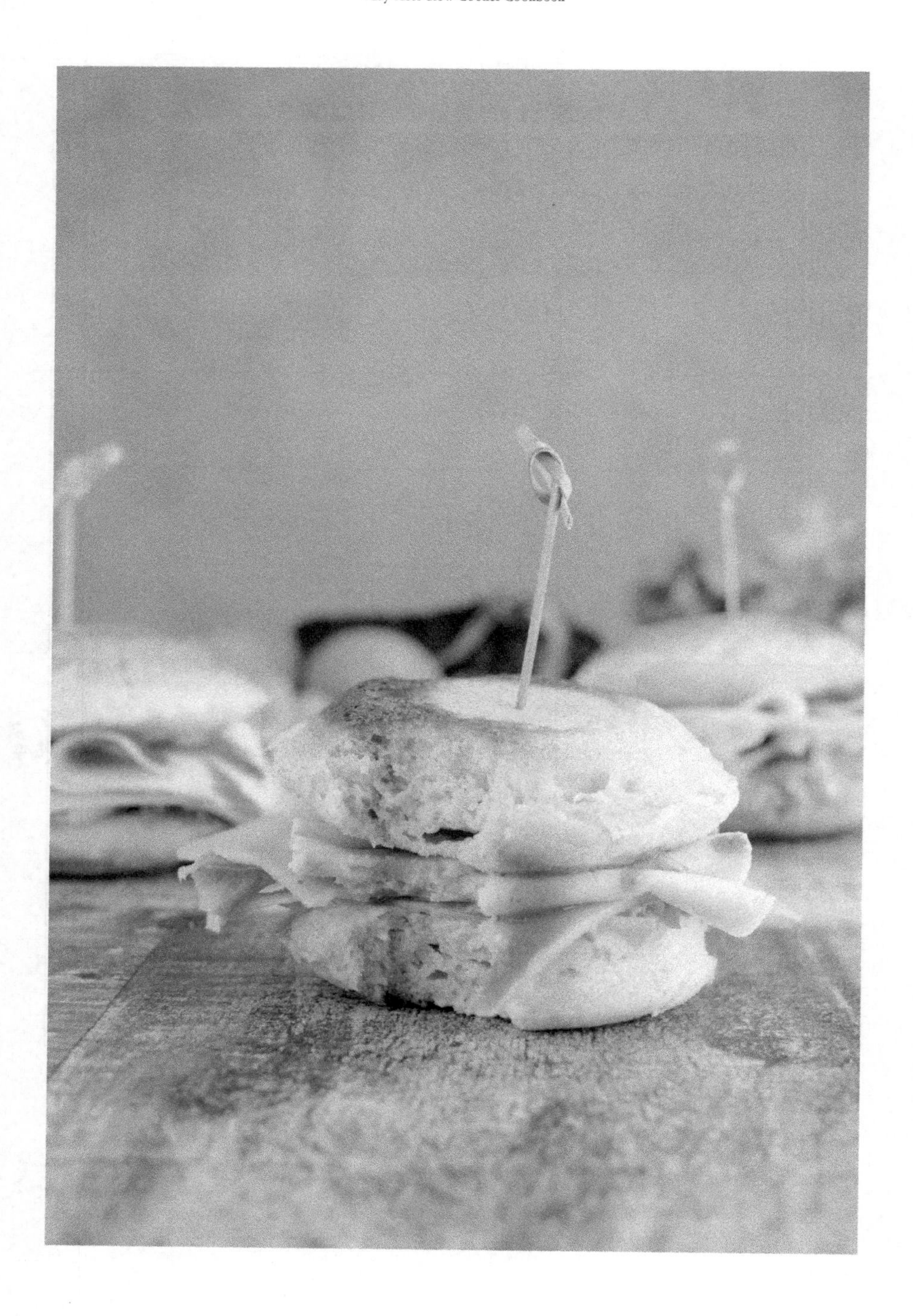

CONCLUSION

Now you can cook healthier meals for yourself, your family, and your friends that will get your metabolism running at the peak of perfection and will help you feel healthy, lose weight, and maintain a healthy balanced diet. A new diet isn't so bad when you have so many options from which to choose. You may miss your carbs, but with all these tasty recipes at your fingertips, you'll find them easily replaced with new favorites.

You will marvel at how much energy you have after sweating though the first week or so of almost no carbs. It can be a challenge, but you can do it! Pretty soon you won't miss those things that bogged down your metabolism as well as your thinking and made you tired and cranky. You will feel like you can rule the world and do anything, once your body is purged of heavy carbs and you start eating things that rejuvenate your body. It is worth the few detox symptoms when you actually start enjoying the food you are eating.

A Keto diet isn't one that you can keep going on and off. It will take your body some time to get adjusted and for ketosis to set in. This process could take anywhere between two to seven days. It is dependent on the level of activity, your body type and the food that you are eating.

There are various mobile applications that you can make use of for tracking your carbohydrate intake. There are paid and free applications as well. These apps will help you in keeping a track of your total carbohydrate and fiber intake. However, you won't be able to track your net carb intake. MyFitnessPal is one of the popular apps. You just need to open the app store on your smartphone, and you can select an app from the various apps that are available.

The amount of weight that you will lose will depend on you. If you add exercise to your daily routine, then the weight loss will be greater. If you cut down on foods that stall weight loss, then this will speed up the process. For instance, completely cutting out things like artificial sweeteners, dairy and wheat products and other related products will definitely help in speeding up your weight loss. During the first two weeks of the Keto diet, you will end up losing all the excess water weight. Ketosis has a diuretic effect on the body, and you might end up losing a couple of pounds within the first few days of this diet. After this, your body will adapt itself to burning fats for generating energy, instead of carbs.

You now have everything you need to break free from a dependence on highly processed foods, with all their dangerous additives that your body interprets as toxins. Today, when you want a sandwich for lunch, you'll roll the meat in Swiss cheese or a lettuce leaf and won't miss the bread at all, unless that is, you've made up the Keto bread recipe you discovered in this book! You can still enjoy your favorite pasta dishes, even taco salad, but without the grogginess in the afternoon that comes with all those unnecessary carbs.

So, energize your life and sustain a healthy body by applying what you've discovered. You don't have to change everything at once. Just start by adopting a new recipe each week that sounds interesting to you. Gradually, swap out less-than-healthy options for ingredients and recipes from this book that will promote your well-being.

Each time you make a healthy substitution or try a new ketogenic recipe, you can feel proud of yourself; you are actually taking good care of your mind and body. Even before you start to experience the benefits of a ketogenic lifestyle, you can feel good because you are choosing the best course for your life.

Thanks for reading.

Lightning Source UK Ltd.
Milton Keynes UK
UKHW020635010321
379583UK00012B/761